CBD Hemp Oil - The Ultimate Guide To CBD and Hemp Oil to Improve Health, Relieve Pain, Reduce Inflammation, And CBD Entrepreneurship

Adidas Wilson

Published by Adidas Wilson, 2021.

While every precaution has been taken in the preparation of this book, the publisher assumes no responsibility for errors or omissions, or for damages resulting from the use of the information contained herein.

CBD HEMP OIL - THE ULTIMATE GUIDE TO CBD AND HEMP OIL TO IMPROVE HEALTH, RELIEVE PAIN, REDUCE INFLAMMATION, AND CBD ENTREPRENEURSHIP

First edition. April 25, 2021.

Copyright © 2021 Adidas Wilson.

ISBN: 979-8201684280

Written by Adidas Wilson.

Disclaimer:

The information contained in this book is intended for educational purposes only and is not a substitute for advice, diagnosis, or treatment by a licensed physician. It is not meant to cover all possible precautions, drug interactions, circumstances, or adverse effects. You should seek prompt medical care for any health issues and consult your doctor before using alternative medicine or making a change to your regimen.

Table of Contents

Introduction

About 4000 years ago, Shen Nung, a Chinese Emperor, and the father of traditional Chinese medicine, believed that hemp could help with absentmindedness, rheumatism, gout issues, and other illnesses. Today, CBD products are not hard to get. They are in boutiques, convenience stores and online stores in the U.S. But even with the widespread use, there is still a lot of misinformation about CBD and how it is derived. What Is CBD? Cannabidiol or CBD is a compound found in the cannabis plant, together with many other cannabinoids, including THC (tetrahydrocannabinol). CBD, unlike marijuana, is extracted from industrial hemp. This is a plant variety that contains less than 0.3% THC. You can obtain a USDA-approved license to cultivate it. The plant does not give the user a "high" and it is believed to have therapeutic and wellness benefits. Consumer interest has been rising steadily since 2016. This could be because of health benefit claims or its association with the cannabis plant. The "breakout" year was 2018, according to EAZE. The number of CBD consumers in the U.S doubled. According to AEZE's data, the most likely consumers of CBD are female baby boomers. They use the products for pain relief, sleep issues, and anxiety. One survey, conducted by Consumer Review, shows that 25% of people in the U.S have tried CBD products in the past two years at least once. This is not hard to believe seeing as CBD is incorporated into many different products in the beauty, beverage, food, and wellness industries. These include lattes, gummies, topicals and tinctures—consumers have a wide range of options. Most CBD users, however, prefer vaping products, according to Brightfield Group. High-CBD flowers are a close second. So, the overall consumer awareness is rising, the interest is growing, and the market growth prospects appear to be solid. Experts have predicted that the CBD retail market will hit $16 billion in the U.S. by 2025. (It was at $2 billion in 2018). 80% of those who know about CBD support its usage—this includes those that do not use it themselves. When you look at these numbers, you realize that an online CBD business can be very lucrative. Hyped products do not usually stick around for long. But CBD is not going anywhere anytime soon if the statistics are anything to go by. If you want to have a piece of the pie, here is how to start an online CBD business. There is a wide range of CBD products: hemp clothes, chewable, creams, accessories, ointments and so many more. So, the first step is deciding what you will sell. Do you want to focus on the classics or trendy stuff? Assess the general niches before you make your decision. The most common ones include - CBD pet products, CBD-based cosmetics, Wellness/supplements products, and CBD-infused beverages/foods. Next, narrow down to product types. These will differ depending on the method of consumption: Sprays and drops: the main ingredients here are CBD oil extracted from hemp and a carrier oil. Sometimes, flavoring agents are included to give the products a pleasant taste and smell. Capsules and pills: a dose of CBD in a soft gel capsule is easier to digest. Most people prefer this method because it is more familiar as well. Cartridges and vapes: recreational users seem to love inhalation products. The same goes for those who like the social aspect of this method. With vaping products, CBD is absorbed faster. So, consumers who are using CBD oil for pain may prefer this method as well. Tinctures: CBD-based tinctures combine cannabinoids with a strong solvent such as alcohol. They may also contain other herbs. Tinctures may not have appealing flavor, but the user will feel the effects quickly. Patches and topicals: these are mainly used for targeted action like menstrual, back, or joint pain. Consumers may also prefer this method if they do not find the hemp flavor appealing. CBD edibles: munchable CBD products include honey sticks, chocolate, candy, and gummies. They make hemp look like more of a treat and less medicinal.

The Farm Bill was passed in 2018. It declared the commercial production of hemp legal in the U.S. It allows for the growing of industrial hemp and legally selling hemp-extracted CBD products across the country. However, there are restrictions: The hemp should contain no more than 0.3% THC. If the THC concentration is higher, it is considered marijuana. 15 states have legalized CBD from marijuana plants for recreational use. 36 states have legalized it for medical use.

Regulations can get a little complicated when it comes to cannabinoids. Epidiolex is the only FDA-approved CBD-based prescription drug. Other CBD brands cannot make health claims as far as their CBD products are concerned. The FDA does not also allow the incorporation of cannabinoids into food. As for the edible CBD products you see on shelves, that is still a gray area. The status of CBD legality is inconsistent across state and federal regulators. FDA does not permit CBD in food, but it also does not act against those selling CBD. They only issue warning letters in case of falsely advertised health claims. Quick recap: Selling federally: CBD selling is legal nationwide according to federal laws. Just make sure the THC level is less than 0.3%. Selling statewide: state laws are different. Industrial hemp-extracted CBD should be allowed. But in states where recreational marijuana is not legal, the restrictions can be unfavorable. Always confirm with a legal specialist. A business plan acts as a guide and it helps you stay up to date with the regulatory policies, new business opportunities and conflicting operational priorities. Besides, your stakeholders and financial supporters will want to see it. Here is what you should include in your CBD business plan: Market analysis: a market analysis provides information about competitors, customers, the industry size, and other variables. Choose a brand name and check the product range: discuss how your brand assets and name set you apart from competition. Explain the CBD niche you are targeting and give a detailed reason why. Talk about your product range briefly. Determine financing: include an estimate of how much you need to get the business going. Break everything down into pre-launch investments and ongoing expenses. Do not forget about unplanned expenses. Include a marketing plan: it shows how you plan to grow awareness, get new customers, and foster repeat purchases. It should be realistic, data-backed, and channel-specific. Here are the two types of licenses you need to start an online CBD business: A business license: register your business with the state. Remember to also ask for an EIN/TIN from the IRS. Reseller license: this is necessary if you plan on buying from wholesalers. Get the certificate from your state. You will not have to pay sales tax when you buy wholesale products. You will also be able to collect sales tax from customers. This is one of the most important steps. If you will be selling your products nationwide, you must make sure that the CBD is derived from industrial hemp and not marijuana. Testing for the THC levels, however, is not cheap. So, buying from a farmer can be challenging. Reputable wholesalers will do the testing and provide COA (certificates of analysis) showing the product's contents. If they cannot do that, it is a huge red flag. Other than product contents, the following are important as well: Pesticide testing, Microbiological testing, and Residual solvents testing. The product's quality is also crucial because it needs to offer the desired effect. CBD production is not regulated. There is no shortage of fake products—some without even a trace of cannabidiol. Do your due diligence so your product does not become one of the fake CBD products. Use the following criteria to assess a potential wholesaler: Extra services (dropshipping, labeling, etc.), Pricing, Reviews from other retailers, Extraction method, Hemp sourcing origin and method, also choose an Ecommerce Platform. You need a good ecommerce platform for your business operations. Here are some great options. BigCommerce: they have lots of B2B and B2C ecommerce tools for CBD manufacturers, wholesalers, and retailers. Shopify: they only allow U.S-based entrepreneurs from specific states to distribute hemp-driven products on the platform. Shift4Shop: they allow entrepreneurs to host their vape and CBD-related businesses. One advantage of an ecommerce platform is that your website development timeline is reduced. Personalize your design: change fonts, layouts, colors, and other important visual elements. Make sure that key information is prominent and digestible. Also, make it easy to navigate the site. Add product descriptions: the information should be fact-based, jargon-free, and devoid of health claims. Upload product pictures: photos influence your customers' purchase decisions, and they are an extension of your business. Come up with a shipping policy: set a threshold for free shipping, determine whether you will have a variable fee, establish a feasible delivery period, and research logistics carriers' policies on CBD products. Pick a shipping solution: shipping and fulfilling software will help you print labels, set shipping rates, auto-dispatch updates to customers and manage logistics. Select a payment processor: most payment processors choose to avoid CBD altogether because it is considered "high-risk". But there are specialized payment processors that handle high-risk businesses. The next step is acquiring customers. Focus on content: there is a lot of misleading content about CBD. Create accurate content about the hemp industry, potential side effects, potential benefits, product types and extraction methods to educate those who are interested. Leverage SEO: well-researched content will help you dominate search engine results. Focus on less-searched long-tail keywords at first. Work with influencers: find a credible advocate who shares the same beliefs and has authority in the CBD niche. If you decide to start a CBD business, prepare to face some unique challenges. Banking and financing: most financial service providers consider CBD a high-risk business. So, opening a merchant account may not be as easy as you expect. The same goes for extra financing. Payment processing: a lot of payment processors will not make life easy for you as a CBD seller. Business insurance: insurers, like banks, are not very accepting. They burden CBD businesses with super-high premiums or bar them altogether. Standing out: there are way too many businesses claiming to sell CBD products. It is not easy to set yourself apart even though your products are genuine and high-quality. Gain customers' trust by positively standing out when it comes to storytelling, accuracy, and transparency. Request for help: with all the complications involved with running a CBD business, it can be overwhelming for a new business owner. Find a mentor who has done this before and let them guide you. Be patient: do not expect an overnight success story. Be patient even as you learn along the way. Know the industry: it seems like every day there are different changes in the industry, moving in contradicting directions. You do not have to change your business based on the latest trends. But make sure you keep up with everything that is going on especially when it comes to compliance requirements and consumer tendencies. A CBD business can be lucrative, but it will not be easy. Do your due diligence before you decide to start your business. Industrial Hemp is now legal, thanks to the 2018 Farm Bill that was signed on December 20 by President Trump. What exactly is "industrial hemp"? It is used to refer to a certain variety of cannabis which, according to the law, has a THC (tetrahydrocannabinol) level of less than 0.3%. THC is the psychoactive compound. This type of cannabis, therefore, cannot get you high. Basically, industrial hemp is no different from any other hardy crop. It does not need a lot of pesticides or chemical fertilizers; it grows fast in most soils and absorbs carbon furiously from the atmosphere. This plant can be used in almost every industry—bioplastics, biofuels, construction materials, textiles, medicines, and foods. The hemp-CBD and cannabis industries are expected to grow to about $42 billion by 2022. So, with this kind of potential, what immediate business opportunities does hemp legalization present? Here are five of the biggest. Cosmetic and nutritional products are expected to be the first to get into the market. People already know that hemp has multiple health benefits. Consumers who practice health and wellness buy a lot of hemp milk, hemp seed oil, hemp seed, and many other products made with hemp. Since CBD products were made legal, they are also buying them—the products are known to treat epilepsy, chronic pain, anxiety, and a host of other conditions. This new freedom, however, is likely to bring new restrictions. The hemp regulatory environment is still being shaped. Farmers and business owners will be required to operate under a structure that has not even been crafted. America is way behind international competition as far as the hemp industry is concerned. Business opportunities are about to start mushrooming because of supply chain gaps. The manufacturing and processing technology being used currently is outdated. The hemp plant is not properly utilized—especially the waste. What gets thrown away is "the real gold". There is a need for the ability to process hemp fully. Most people think that CBD is a huge part of the wellness benefits of hemp. However, CBD is a category on its own. There is still more research to be done but it has been suggested that CBD can treat multiple conditions. It is usually in oil form and can be applied topically, vaped, or infused into drink and food. In some small hometowns, the local farmers have been trying for a while to increase their revenue. Even jobs have become scarce with some industries closing. Hemp can turn this situation around. It is a product that moves quickly. This will be amazing for farmers with little storage capacity. Consumers are excited about using hemp as a raw material. Companies are already using hemp to make clothing. There is also the dramatic opportunity of using hemp—either alone or combined with other plants such as corn—to make bioplastics that are compostable. Hemp is a plant with a myriad of benefits. To show you its true potential, the following is an extensive list of products that you can try.

Foods & Drinks

Hemp seeds: these are superfoods like chia and flax seeds.

Hemp seed oil

Protein powder: this is a vegetarian protein, popular among athletes.

Hemp tea

Energy bars: these are filled with high-quality ingredients for a quality snack.

Hemp coffee

Hemp veggie burgers

Hemp herbal flavored water

Hemp seed butter

Hemp milk

Hemp vodka

Hemp beer

Hemp hot dogs

Hemp flour: nutritious and gluten-free.

Hemp granola: easy to make at home.

Clothing and Accessories

Hemp fabric is superior in that it is more: eco-friendly, durable, and breathable.

Shirts

Jeans: hemp jeans are absorbent and have microbial properties.

Hemp shoes

Hemp coat/jacket: you can find a wide variety of these at Hood lamb.

Backpacks

Yoga pants

Sunglasses

Hats: check out Tin lid Hats for cool hemp hats.

Hemp beanie

Wallets

Hemp socks: these are way better than cotton.

Totes

Flip flops (sandals)

Belts

Scarfs: they are cozy, warm, and lightweight.

Bow ties and ties.

Pocket squares and handkerchiefs

Bracelets

Robes

Overalls

Beauty & Skin

Hemp skin care products are superior to conventional products. Here are a few that you should try.

Body lotions: they are great for people with skin conditions.

Lip Balms

Conditioner and shampoo

Body wash: hemp soaps are less drying and smoother than traditional soaps.

Facial cleanser and cream: hemp oils are best for people with sensitive skin.

Hemp sunscreen

Hemp serum

Health

Hemp extract (CBD)

Hemp essential oil

Soothing aromatherapy candles: these are made using hemp essential oil. They help you relax.

Massage oil

Hemp heat muscle rub: CBD (Cannabidiol) helps with arthritis and joint pains.

Vape juice.

Pets

Dog toys: hemp toys are durable.

Dog collar & leash: your dog cannot chew through it.

Animal bedding

Pet tinctures (CBD oil for dogs)

Automobiles

Sports cars

Biofuel: cars that use regular fuel can use hemp biofuel, no need for new cars.

Thermoset compression molding

Home and Office

Pens: you can engrave a personal message on hemp pens made by Green Spring Technologies.

Hemp sheets

Hemp towel

Paper

Hemp curtains

Laundry detergent: it works like normal detergent except it is hypoallergenic and non-toxic.

Hemp crafts

Hemp chair

Tablecloths

Hemp blankets: they are breathable and perfect for summer. They are also ideal for people with skin conditions.

Farming and Gardening

Hemp growing mats.

Soil cleanup: hemp has deep roots that stabilize the structure of soil.

Industrial and Others

Ropes

Plastics: hemp plastic is more sustainable and durable.

Building homes – hempcrete

Oil spill cleanup

Hemp flags: hemp makes rustic, durable flags. Hemp batteries: hemp fibers are way more conducive compared to graphene. It is, therefore, a great source of batteries and supercapacitors. There are thousands of ways in which hemp can be used. Being eco-friendly and sustainable this is just the beginning. Legalization comes with numerous opportunities, some of which many people did not even expect. Cannabis oil is among the biggest expansion areas. Cannabis oil has different meanings, but the most important thing is that it offers entrepreneurs and consumers a new way of exploring and benefitting from the blooming marijuana industry. What makes cannabis oil a big industry? How can entrepreneurs get a piece of the pie? Cannabis oil comes in different types. Each one of them is famous and keeps increasing in popularity. The Brightfield Group says that the CBD market is expected to reach $22 billion by 2022. Cannabis oil is more than just CBD. THC-rich waxes and concentrates are oils too, technically. The sale of recreational cannabis concentrates is predicted to get to $8.5 billion in 2022. Cannabis oil, in some cases, is a kind of concentrate high in tetrahydrocannabinol (THC). This is the weed compound that makes you feel high. Usually, oil rich in THC is vaped. Other forms of high THC concentrates are resin, shatter, and wax. All these concentrates are getting popular by the day. A survey was carried out among California cannabis users and it was found that vaping is one of the most popular delivery methods for both old and young consumers. This is due to a few reasons: It is safer compared to dry herbs. During the cannabis oil extraction process, all the bacteria is killed. Vaping is much more discreet and convenient. A vapor is easier to carry everywhere. The oil contains consistent CDB and THC levels, unlike flowers. Therefore, you will get a steadier high. Oil is more concentrated and guarantees a stronger high. As a caution, always be careful and follow instructions for vaping tools. Cannabis oil is not just used as a recreational concentrate. CBD (Cannabidiol) is among the fastest growing forms of concentrates. It cannot get you high. CBD is the key non-psychoactive compound in hemp and marijuana. Unlike THC, it interacts with the body differently and does not give a "high". It has significant medicinal and medical benefits. It reduces inflammation, anxiety, acne, pain, and even seizures in epileptic people. It can also be efficient in preventing arthritis and neurodegenerative diseases such as Parkinson's and Alzheimer's. Cannabis oil may be popular, but it is still an undeveloped market when it comes to production. Both CBD and THC oil are extracted using the same kind of equipment. To extract cannabis oil, you need a lot of equipment and expertise in that area. It can be done in one of two ways: Solvent extraction and Carbon dioxide (CO2) extraction. Join the extraction business: after flower, vape is the second biggest product category. Your extraction business will face the same issues that all other weed companies face. Create a CBD company: CBD may become a global market very soon because of its medicinal and medical uses. A clear standard has not yet been established as far as branding cannabis is concerned. This makes the process both thrilling and challenging. Up until several years ago, packaging was not a relevant thought to many manufacturers. In the past, you could not find cannabis displayed in retail stores and cannabis dispensaries. People passed it in bags without labels. As you learn more about this industry, you will realize that packaging must sensitively balance progressive transparency, safety, consumer education and aesthetic appeal. If you are involved in branding cannabis, you must stay updated with the budtender and consumer evolution along with any new state regulations. What does the consumer know? Is there something you should teach them? What measures can you take to make sure that they consume the product properly? All these are public concerns, and your clients will bring related problems to you. Before you begin, know that there are a few things that you need to incorporate. The laws of the state will have a huge influence on this. Here is important information that should be on your label. Understand harvest dates, it is not uncommon for cultivators to deliver to you a full-price flower that is a year or more past the harvest dates. Even though the flower tested at 25% (according to them), understand that after a year THC loses potency. The flower may burn before it is smoked if it is too dry. Therefore, your packaging should always include the harvesting date. A buyer cannot know how much flower there is just by looking. Depending on strain, a gram may appear smaller or larger. It all depends on the density of the buds. Some buyers are first-time consumers and including the quantity makes them more confident. They will know that they are buying the right number of edibles, concentrate or flower. Individuals respond differently to cannabinoids. Many cannabis brands list CBD and THC percentages because these cannabinoids are well understood in the industry. What many do not know is that there are 113 identified cannabinoids so far. CBD and THC may be the most abundant, but it is still important to test for extra cannabinoids and if any is 0.5%+, it should be listed. The number of terpenes in cannabis is still unknown. According to research, terpenes dictate how high you will get, the flavor of the bud and the aroma. Include the terpene profile on your label to help the consumer get a strain that matches their preferences. For medical cannabis, the pesticides used in cultivation matter. Most customers prefer pesticide-free or natural pesticides options. Have this information on the label so they know what they are getting. Quite a few recreational users may also be skeptical in this area. Some states require that the Unified Business Identifier (UBI) of the testing lab be included on the packaging. Even if it is not required in your state, be sure to include it alongside the processor and/or producer.

Chapter One
Hemp Seed Oil and CBD Oil

Ever since the Food and Drug Administration approved the first CBD-based drug, people have become more curious about the benefits of CBD and hemp seed oils. A lot of consumers get confused by these names though. Hemp oil is another name for CBD oil. Some people tend to think that hemp seed oil is the same as hemp oil. But CBD oil and hemp seed oil are two different products. CBD oil is produced using the flowers, leaves and stalks of the hemp plant. These parts have a high CBD concentration—a compound that has many potential health benefits. Hemp seed oil, on the other hand, comes from the Cannabis sativa plant seeds. The seeds have no CBD. However, they are rich in fatty acids and other nutrients as well as useful bioactive compounds. Understanding CBD oil and hemp seed oil will help consumers and clinicians choose the most appropriate and safest product. So, here is all you need to know about the two products. Hemp seed oil is derived from the Cannabis sativa plant seeds. It contains gamma-linolenic acid, omega-3 fatty acids, omega-6 fatty acids, among other nutritional antioxidants. It also contains high levels of Vitamin D and B. Hemp seed oil cannot get you high since it contains little to no CBD and no THC (tetrahydrocannabinol) at all. Hemp seed oil can be used for recreational purposes. It contains little or no CBD and THC—the compounds that have psychoactive effects. Hemp seed oil may be found in some nutritional supplements due to the high levels of nutrients. Hemp seed oil may be used in the manufacture of fibers and clothing. Some believe that hemp seed oil is good for cardiovascular health because it improves: Triglycerides, Low-density lipoprotein cholesterol

High-density lipoprotein cholesterol

Total cholesterol

More research is still being conducted on these claims.

Effects and Benefits

Hemp seed oil is added to nutritional products because it contains high levels of essential amino acids and unsaturated fatty acids.

Other possible benefits of hemp seed oil include:

Improving gastrointestinal health

Improving skin conditions

Boosting the immune system

Better cardiovascular health

Anti-cancer effects

Anti-aging effects

How It Is Made

Hemp seed oil is extracted from the hemp plant seeds.

Risks and Side Effects

Hemp seed oil is safe.

It may not help with cardiovascular health.

Getting high is unlikely.

CBD Oil

There are three different kinds of CBD oil.

Full-spectrum CBD oil (it contains all cannabis compounds including THC, but in low levels).

Broad-spectrum CBD oil (contains some of the compounds, no THC).

CBD oil (it only contains CBD and is made using CBD isolate).

Check the COA (Certificate of Analysis) to know what you are buying.

Uses

CBD-derived products are believed to help with:

Neurodegenerative conditions

Inflammatory skin conditions

Addiction management

Depression and anxiety

Inflammation and pain

Epilepsy

All these benefits, apart from antiepileptic benefits, need to be researched further.

CBD oils with THC can be used for recreational purposes.

It is also possible that these oils contain terpenoids and Phyto cannabinoids in small amounts.

How It Works

Research is still being conducted on this. But it is possible that CBD:

Inhibits endocannabinoid reuptake.

Activates the transient receptor potential vanilloid.

Makes serotonin receptors more active.

Effects and Benefits

There are different components in CBD oils, and they all have their benefits.

CBD has neuroprotective, antidepressant, antiepileptic, antianxiety, and anti-inflammatory effects.

How It Is Made

CBD oil is extracted from the leaves and flowers of the plant.

Risks and Side Effects

CBD-derived products are generally safe with minimal side effects. Just make sure you can trust your source.

Chapter Two
Beginner's Guide to CBD

CBD (Cannabidiol) oil is produced from the cannabis plant. Although it is believed to have health benefits, it comes with risks and is illegal in some states. The FDA (Food and Drug Administration) approved the use of Epidiolex in June 2018 for treating epilepsy. Other states have legalized some forms of cannabis. Cannabis comprises a wide variety of compounds and they all have different effects. Some can be used for medical purposes. What Is CBD Oil? CBD is a cannabinoid or compound (one of many) found in the cannabis plant. There is research being conducted to determine its possible therapeutic uses. Marijuana contains two compounds: CBD and delta-9 tetrahydrocannabinol. Both compounds will affect you differently. THC used to be the most popular compound in cannabis. It has psychological effects and is the most active. When ingested or smoked, it gives a "high". CBD, on the other hand, is not psychoactive. While it will not change your state of mind, it can cause changes in your body and may have health benefits. Where Do You Get CBD from? It is extracted from the cannabis plant, also known as marijuana or the hemp plant (depending on the THC levels). Hemp plants with less than 0.3% THC are legal. All cannabinoids interact with cannabinoid receptors (part of the endocannabinoid system) to produce effects in your body. There are two receptors produced by the body: CB1 receptors: they are found throughout the body, especially in the brain. These are responsible for coordinating movement, appetite, thinking, mood, emotion, pain, memories, etc. CB2 receptors: these are commonly found in the immune system. The receptors affect pain and inflammation. CBD stimulates the receptors, prompting the body to produce its own cannabinoids (endocannabinoids). THC will attach to CB1. People take CBD oil for the following reasons: Lung conditions, Multiple sclerosis (MS), Epilepsy and seizure disorders, Asthma or allergies, Cancer, Nausea, PTSD, Migraine, Sleep disorder, Depression and anxiety, Joint pain or arthritis, Chronic pain, Acne, Type 1 diabetes, Parkinson's disease, and Alzheimer's disease, some of these claims are backed by scientific research. Anti-Inflammatory and Natural Pain Relief Properties - There is some evidence showing that CBD and other non-psychoactive compounds can treat chronic pain. A few studies have shown that CBD reduces nicotine cravings. Epidiolex is a purified form of CBD and the FDA approved it for treatment of Dravet Syndrome and Lennox-Gastaut Syndrome for patients aged 3 and over. Some studies show that CBD can slow down the onset of Alzheimer's. A 2012 study revealed that CBD can have the same effects as antipsychotic drugs. CBD can help in curbing the spread of certain types of cancer. Hemp and hemp products with a THC level below 0.3% are legal under the Farm Bill. But be sure to confirm with your state laws. CBD has its risks. It does not help that most CBD products have not been approved by the FDA. To be on the safe side, speak to a doctor first. How to Use CBD - Mixing with drink or food, By use of a dropper or pipette, In capsules, Massaging into skin, and Spraying under the tongue. Many countries are now legalizing cannabidiol (CBD) products and this has led to an increase in the number of consumers. One of the methods people use to ingest the compound is through vaping. There are studies supporting claims that CBD helps with chronic conditions such as pain and anxiety. But most of these studies are based on people taking CBD orally—not by inhaling it. The CDC advises against vaping because its long-term effects are still not known. Here is all you need to know about CBD vaping. What Is CBD? CBD is extracted from cannabis. It does not make the user high, like THC (tetrahydrocannabinol). People use CBD for the following potential effects: Epilepsy and seizure treatment, Anti-anxiety, Anti-inflammation, and Pain relief. Researchers are also looking into how CBD can help with anxiety disorder, some childhood diseases, and neurodegenerative diseases. The FDA approved Epidiolex, a CBD-containing solution, to be used in treating some forms of epilepsy. Doctors in Europe and Canada can prescribe Sativex in the treatment of spasticity. The main challenge, for both doctors and consumers, is that there are no standardized dosages. Vaping CBD Oil - People have started using e-cigarettes for marijuana products. There are not enough studies on CBD oil vaping. Most CBD clinical trials mainly focus on oral solutions, sublingual sprays and oral capsules. Aerosolized therapies are used for people with chronic obstructive pulmonary disease and asthma. The therapies have a rapid clinical effect. But with vaping, researchers are still studying its risks and benefits. Risks of CBD Vaping - CBD derived from *Cannabis sativa* has still not been approved by the FDA for medicinal use. The labeling and manufacturing of CBD products is also not regulated. Vape pens can offer an effective method of delivering drugs into the system. But most CBD products are not correctly labelled. People can easily be exposed to unknown CBD doses and other dangerous components. There have been recent cases of people who have suffered severe lung injury due to vaping. Some of those people died as a result. The CDC recommends the following for those who vape: Avoid THC-containing vaping products or e-cigarettes from shady sources. Avoid vaping products or e-cigarettes with vitamin E acetate. Avoid adding extra ingredients to your vaping products. Do not use vaping products and e-cigarettes if you are a young adult or pregnant. Always buy pens and formulations from reliable sources. The FDA does not regulate these products so finding the right one can be a challenge. Most people take cannabis for pain. But there are still no clear studies showing the effect of CBD vaping on pain. CBD for Depression - People use cannabis for depression, anxiety, and pain. But most studies do not show how a consistent use of CBD affects depression. Some studies show that chronic cannabis usage could make depressive symptoms worse. So far, scientific studies indicate that CBD could help with: Post-traumatic stress disorder. Obsessive-compulsive disorder. Social anxiety disorder. Panic disorder. and generalized anxiety disorder. Note: there are still no dosing guidelines and most of these studies focused on oral cannabis intake.

Chapter Three
How to Take CBD

Cannabis plants contain many different types of cannabinoids. Scientists are still trying to research them all. So far, there is one that looks promising as far as health benefits go. CBD or cannabidiol is non intoxicating, unlike THC (tetrahydrocannabinol). You will not get high when you use it. Research about this compound is still ongoing and it is not regulated by the FDA. It has only been approved for treatment of epilepsy. Some studies have shown that it can help with nerve damage, inflammation, and Alzheimer's. What to Look for in a CBD Product - Broad- or Full-Spectrum - You want products that are made using broad or full spectrum oils and not isolate or distillate. Full-spectrum oils have all the cannabinoids, including THC. Broad-spectrum oils have most compounds, but generally no THC. Look for products that have been tested by a third-party lab. U.S-Grown, Organic - There are agricultural regulations in the U.S. Edibles such as mints, gummies or truffles mask the "weedy" taste. Research, however, shows that it may take up to two hours for the edible to kick in and you only absorb 20 to 30 percent. This is due to the "first pass effect". Most edibles will contain preservatives and sugars. If you do not want any of these, a sublingual product may be best for you. You absorb them under your tongue. The products include lozenges, oils, sprays, and tinctures. This is better than eating edibles because the product is not subjected to the digestive tract. Most of the CBD will be preserved. CBD topicals are applied to the skin directly. There are CBD-infused transdermal patches, salves, creams, balms, and lotions. If the skin condition or pain is localized, topicals are a good option. A 2015 study showed that applying CBD gel on the skin can reduce joint swelling. It was done on rats, but the results are promising for people with arthritis. Research on topicals is still ongoing. But this is what is known so far: There is no first pass effect with topicals. They offer concentrated relief. Your skin has poor permeability. So, you may want to get a product with a high concentration of CBD. Vaping and Smoking - You can inhale CBD concentrates (like sugar waxes) using a vaping pen, use a vaporizer with a CBD oil cartridge or smoke the cannabis flower as a joint. When you smoke or vape, the CBD goes into your bloodstream directly. The effects will come faster, compared to other methods. You can absorb 34% to 56% within 10 minutes or even less. You should know that smoking CBD may expose someone to carcinogens. Vaping may reduce this risk, but it is still not clear how safe it is. If you opt for vaping, do not use cartridges made with carriers or thinning agents—think vegetable glycerin, propylene glycol or fractionated coconut oil. These compounds can be harmful to lung tissue. To find the perfect method for you, you must try different CBD products and make your decision. But talk to your doctor before you start trying.

Chapter Four
Choosing a CBD Oil

CBD or cannabidiol oil is extracted from the cannabis plant. The oil has therapeutic benefits and is believed to treat cancer, epilepsy, and anxiety. Most CBD products contain low levels of THC (tetrahydrocannabinol), the main psychoactive cannabinoid, so you will not get high. You will find very many CBD tinctures and oils in the market, but they are not all the same. None of the OTC CBD products have been approved by the FDA. Some of them may not be effective or reliable. The ones listed here are: Meant for oral consumption. Third-party tested. Extracted from U.S-grown hemp. Full spectrum (THC levels are below 0.3%). The Best CBD Oils. Charlotte's Web CBD Oil. CBD type: full spectrum. CBD potency: 210 to 18,000 mg per 30ml bottle. COA: available online. The brand that makes this one is well known. And for the potency, their prices are fair. It is made using coconut oil, hemp extract and flavorings. Natural Cannabis Full-Spectrum CBD Drops. CBD type: full spectrum - CBD potency: 300 to 6,000 mg per 30ml to 120ml bottle - COA: available on the product page. They use organic cannabis, sourced from U.S farms. This product is hemp-oil based and THC-free. You can get it in different flavors, sizes, and strengths. Natural products are affordable. This oil may be labelled as "full-spectrum" but it is actually "isolate" because it contains CBD only—no other cannabinoids. NuLeaf Naturals Full-Spectrum CBD Oil - CBD type: full spectrum - CBD potency: 1,800 mg per 30ml bottle. COA: available online - This one is highly concentrated. The company grows hemp plants in Colorado. Holmes Organics CBD Oil Tincture

CBD type: broad-spectrum. CBD potency: 450 to 900 mg per 30ml bottle. COA: available online. All products from Holmes Organics are THC-free, U.S-sourced and lab-tested. Absolute Nature CBD Full-Spectrum CBD Oil Drops. CBD type: full spectrum. CBD potency: 500 to 1,000 mg per 30ml bottle. COA: available online. The product is made using non-GMO hemp from Colorado. Veritas Farms Full Spectrum CBD Tincture. CBD type: full spectrum. CBD potency: 250 to 2000 mg per 30ml bottle. COA: available online. This one is also made using non-GMO hemp from Colorado. Lazarus Naturals High Potency CBD Tincture. CBD type: full spectrum. CBD potency: 750 mg per 15ml bottle, 3,000 mg per 60ml bottle or 6,000 mg per 120ml bottle. COA: available on the product page. The hemp used to make this oil is from Oregon. The company is transparent about the entire process. Ojai Energetics Full Spectrum Hemp Elixir. CBD type: full spectrum. CBD potency: 250 mg per 30ml bottle. COA: available online. It does not contain any synthetically modified compounds. CBD Distillery Full-Spectrum CBD Oil. Tincture oil contains up to 167 mg per serving. They use non-GMO hemp. 4 Corners Cannabis Oral Tincture. CBD type: full spectrum. CBD potency: 250 to 500 mg per 15ml bottle. COA: available online. 4 Corners oil contains over 60% CBD. You can mix it with your drink or take it on its own. How to Choose a CBD Oil or Tincture. Here are the factors to consider: Type of CBD in the product. Whether it has been tested by a third-party. Any other ingredients in the product. Where the cannabis is grown (and whether it is organic).

Chapter Five
CBD Dosage

People keep talking about CBD and its health benefits. But how much product should you consume to experience the benefits? The cannabis plant has more than 60 active compounds and CBD or cannabidiol is one of them. The active compounds, or cannabinoids, all have different effects on the human body. CBD will not get you high as it is not psychoactive. Scientific research has shown that it could help with: IBD (inflammatory bowel disease) Heart health, Inflammation and pain, seizure for epilepsy patients, sleep, and depression and anxiety. Regardless of what you want to treat, you must figure out the correct dosage—otherwise, it may not work. CBD is not regulated by the FDA, so knowing how much to take can be tricky. But this guide can help. People have researched and talked a lot about CBD over the recent years. A 2017 review shows that CBD is relatively safe, according to research. However, the studies do not give a universal dosage amount. The review points out that people will respond differently to varying dosages. In most of the studies where humans were the subjects, they used 20 to 1,500 mg of CBD per day. There is still a lot of research to be done on CBD. How Much Should You Take? The answer to this question depends on several factors. They include: The CBD concentration in a gummy, drop, capsule or pill. Simply put, the decision on how much to take depends on several variables. You should always consult your doctor for potential risks and appropriate dosage. This is especially important especially if you are taking CBD prescription medication like Epidiolex. If you do not get a recommendation from your doctor, you may want to start small. This could be 20 to 40 mg a day and increase it gradually (like

5 mg a week). Keep increasing until you find the dosage amount that treats your symptoms. Keep track of the dosages and how you feel. CBD products like pills, capsules and gummies will show how much is in a serving. In the case of a bottle of CBD capsules, for instance, the packaging may show that a capsule contains 5 mg of CBD. CBD oil mainly comes in a dropper bottle. The manufacturer might indicate on the packaging the amount of CBD in one drop. Other manufacturers will only indicate how much CBD is in the entire bottle. You will have to calculate the amount in a single drop. One drop $\approx$ 0.05 ml. Is There Anything Like Too Much CBD? A 2011 review showed that the human body handles continued CBD use well—even with a dose as high as 1,500 mg a day. A 2017 update confirmed it. A 2019 study, however, raised concerns about potential damage to the liver. The study was done on mice. Known side effects of CBD may include fatigue, appetite changes and diarrhea. Note: beware of low-quality and fake CBD products. Consult Your Doctor - Before you try any CBD product, it is best to see your doctor first.

Chapter Six
How to Read a CBD Label

This is a good time to shop for CBD products. But as a consumer, you must be very observant while reading the labels—regardless of whether you are shopping in a licensed store, over the counter, or online. You must know exactly what you are buying. If you want to be fluent in the CBD label language, keep reading. CBD Label Requirements - Different states have different requirements for CBD products labels. The strongest requirements come in medical cannabis systems and state-licensed programs. There are still no federal regulations for CBD. However, most CBD manufacturers mimic the appearance of federal dietary labels. Questionable CBD products have labels that do not look like mainstream food labels or state-licensed products. CBD Dosage - The label on a product can tell you a lot about CBD dosage—the serving size, number of servings, milligrams of CBD per serving and even the total milligrams in the entire package. Note: some CBD labels can be inaccurate. CBD Milligrams - Every CBD product in the market should state how much CBD is contained in the package (in milligrams). Servings Per Container and Servings Size - The number of servings in a container and the milligrams of CBD in a single serving is also important information. A serving size lets you know what is meant by one serving. One good example of a serving size is one gummy bear. And if one gummy bear contains 10 mg of CBD, that is the amount per serving. The number of servings in this case would be the number of gummy bears in a container. CBD Oil Source - It is good to know where your CBD comes from. The CBD products you see in the adult-use and medical cannabis markets are sourced from plants which are bred for their strong flavors, aromas and effects. They contain THC, the psychoactive cannabinoid. Hemp-derived CBD, on the other hand, is found in industrial hemp plants. Their THC level is less than 0.3%. You should also know about the following: Full spectrum CBD - contains other terpenes and cannabinoids, including THC. Broad-spectrum CBD: contains other terpenes and cannabinoids, but no THC. CBD isolate: this one contains almost pure CBD crystals. Red flag: watch out for labels that barely mention CBD. They, instead, use phrases like "hemp oil" or "hemp extract". What to Look Out for - Batch and Lot Number - Batch and lot numbers are mandated by advanced medical or state-licensed adult-use cannabis systems. It shows accountability and helps with regulation. Manufacturing Date - CBD, like most products, degrades over time. It is important to know the age of the product. License Number - State-licensed manufacturers must indicate their license number. It should be on the label. Third-party certification confirms the claims by the manufacturer. Other Ingredients - Most CBD products include other non-CBD products like flavors and glycerin. QR codes are not mandatory but they assure quality. Read and adhere to the disclaimers and warnings. Contact information such as the company's website should be included on the label. Ingredients to Avoid - Vague terms ("hemp extract", "hemp oil" "natural ingredients") Essential oils, vitamins, flavorings thickeners, vegetable oil, thinners, and other additives in vape pens.

Chapter Seven
CBD and Cannabis for Pets

More and more pet owners are giving cannabis-derived products to their pets to help with conditions such as seizures and pain. These products have high CBD levels and low THC levels. But has scientific research been done to determine the effects of cannabinoid medicine on pets? Yes, but not much. So far, the issue of using medical cannabis to help with the health of a cat or dog is still complicated. You will not find sufficient peer-reviewed research showing its effectiveness or safety. A leading international journal, Frontiers in Veterinary Science, published the first clinical study on this subject in 2018. The study sought to determine the effect that hemp-based cannabidiol would have on arthritic dogs. The findings were encouraging. Over 80% of the dog subjects showed significant improvement in mobility and decrease in pain. But a single study is not enough. Unfortunately, there are not many other studies. There is still a lot to learn. Regardless of what the professional or opinion of a vet is, most states do not allow Vets to recommend or prescribe cannabis for your pet. This even applies in California where cannabis is legal for adults. Dr. Gary Richter, an Oakland-based veterinarian, started an online petition for an animals' "compassionate care" law. An almost similar bill was passed in the state. Vets still cannot recommend cannabis without risking their licenses. The situation gets even tougher in states that have not legalized cannabis for any kind of use. This makes it difficult for researchers. Some scientists have managed to publish peer-reviewed work, despite the restrictions. There has been a lot of discussion surrounding the toxicity of marijuana to animals. That is, when pets accidentally eat the owner's supply. And a

2004 study proved that marijuana poisoning in dogs is possible. This study was based on an mg per kg dosage. Most of the studies done in the 2000s confirmed the mild toxicity of the plant. The recent study on dogs with arthritis has allowed scientists to have a deeper understanding of cannabis and how it works in an animal's body. Previously, CBD was given to dogs in the form of pills and the absorption was poor. Oil absorption has proven to be much better. Dr. Joseph Wakshlag (of the 2018 study) settled on 2 mg per kg body weight. A couple of successful human studies have used 1 – 5 mg. So, they decided to settle somewhere between that. THC is toxic for dogs. But some experts, like Richter, believe that it can be beneficial to animals. Dr. Richter advises pet owners to do their own research and see whether THC can help their pets. Richter says that cannabis has helped his own dog, Leo, with seizures. And Colorado State University has a promising study underway to confirm this. What About Cats? Cats respond differently and there is extraordinarily little research on cannabis for cats. ElleVet has two studies underway for cats: one for chronic UTIs and another one for pain.

Chapter Eight
Myths and Controversies

Everyone seems to be interested in cannabidiol (CBD). There is a lot of information everywhere you turn—but it is not all accurate. CBD is incredibly therapeutic and safe but there are so many myths surrounding it. Here are the most common ones. Myth 1: CBD Is Medical and Non-Psychoactive While THC Is Recreational. Many articles and even scientific papers term CBD as non-psychoactive. This implies that it does not affect one's consciousness. But how can this be, yet CBD has proven to have mood-elevating, anti-craving, anti-psychoactive and anti-anxiety effects on humans? Clearly, CBD impacts your psyche, but in a beneficial way. It is, however, non-intoxicating and non-impairing. THC has also shown to have many medicinal properties. Myth 2: CBD Has a Sedating Effect. CBD, on its own, is not sedating. If anything, it is alerting. It delays sleep time, reduces THC hangovers, and generally counters THC sedative effects. Even in high does, think 600 mg in one dose, CBD does not have a sedating effect. Some varieties of high-CBD cannabis may contain a sedating terpene. Myth 3: CBD Is Enough in Small Doses. CBD, compared to THC, is less potent when it comes to relieving symptoms. With pain or anxiety, you may require only 3 to 5 mg of THC. But with CBD, you may require from 30 to 200 mg for the same results. This is not to say that CBD is not beneficial in small doses. Myth 4: CBD Is the Same. A CBD molecule from the laboratory is no different from one sourced from hemp or medical cannabis. But the various CBD products you see on the market do not have the same effect. CBD works best alongside other cannabinoids (compounds in the cannabis plant), especially THC. CBD has therapeutic effects while THC will reduce its adverse effects. And this is the case even when the THC level is extremely low. The difference between hemp and medical cannabis can seem blurry at times. But so far, it appears that hemp is not a very efficient source of CBD. If possible, always go for lab-tested, locally grown, and artisanal produced CBD products. This may mean that you must buy from a state-licensed retailer. Myth 5: CBD Activates Cannabinoid Receptors. Everyone has an endocannabinoid system. It helps in restoring balance as well as responding to injury and illness. It is always working to keep you healthy. This system is, therefore, mostly targeted for therapeutic interventions. But CBD does not stimulate CB2 or CB1 receptors. It reduces their activity level, reducing the THC effects. It also increases cannabinoid signaling indirectly. The science of cannabinoids is filled with paradoxes and opposites which can be hard to understand. Myth 6: CBD Is legal Everywhere in the United States. CBD is widely available almost everywhere—at your local tobacco shop, health food store and even on Amazon. This has led many people to think that it is legal. But the DEA will strongly disagree on that. People started using CBD even before the pandemic to relieve anxiety, inflammation, pain and stress. The good thing is that it doesn't cause the "high" which can make the use of cannabis for treatment complicated.

However, CBD has many other health benefits. And if you are a woman, you may consider incorporating it into your lifestyle. According to research, CBD can provide solutions to various women's health issues such as sleep disorders, sexual performance, hormonal imbalances, stress, and anxiety. Here are three amazing CBD benefits for women and how to effectively use the product. But before that... What Is CBD? Cannabidiol, or CBD, is an active compound that occurs naturally in the cannabis (also known as hemp or marijuana) plant. The cannabis sativa plant has more than 80 cannabinoids. But THC (the psychoactive compound) and CBD are the most popular cannabinoids. CBD is not psychoactive so it will not give you a "high" like THC. Additionally,

CBD oil usually contains less than 0.3% THC (the legal amount) so it cannot get you high. Clinical trials continue to confirm the effectiveness of CBD. FDA ever approved a CBD-containing drug for pediatric seizures, Epidiolex. So, here is how CBD can be beneficial for women's health.

CBD Helps with Sexual Performance - Some evidence suggests that couples who are regular cannabis users have more sex. However, THC can have unwanted effects like dry mouth while kissing, feeling overwhelmed or being "too high".

The good thing about CBD is that you get the positive cannabis effects without the negative THC effects. The female reproductive system has cannabinoid receptors all over—the vulva, vagina, ovaries, fallopian tubes, and the uterus. These receptors play an important role when it comes to the pain or pleasure associated with sex. These receptors can help with achieving orgasms and low libido. CBD increases nerve sensation and blood flow which may translate to intense orgasms and sexual pleasure. Using CBD for Better Sex - Get a CBD salve massage from your partner to help you relax. Have a CBD bath together with your partner beforehand? Take a few drops of CBD oil about 30 minutes before sex. CBD Can Help with Menstrual Cramps - Periods come with a lot of annoying symptoms like headaches, mood swings, bloating, cramps, etc. Non-Steroidal Anti-Inflammatory Drugs (NSAIDs) inhibit the enzymes that produce prostaglandins. But they also have a lot of side effects. CBD, on the other hand, offers anti-inflammatory benefits, but without all those side effects. Using CBD for Menstrual Cramps Relief - Get a warm CBD bath soak for roughly 20 minutes. Use a CBD salve or oil to massage wherever you are feeling the pain. Take CBD dark chocolate. CBD Can Help with Menopause Symptoms - The transition to menopause can come with depression, anxiety, sleeplessness, and mood swings. Several studies show that CBD can be beneficial to women transitioning to menopause. Using CBD for Menopause - Use a topical CBD salve for pain, tense muscles, and inflammation. Try CBD oil for stress and anxiety. Take a warm CBD bath before bed. CBD or cannabidiol is among the many cannabinoids found in the marijuana and hemp plants. For a long time, CBD has been in the shadow of THC (tetrahydrocannabinol), the intoxicating cannabinoid. CBD has recently started becoming more popular than THC. Most experts consider it safe as it relieves pain, boosts mood and induces calm, without giving a high. So far, research shows that CBD could have many great health benefits. But researchers are worrying about false claims that seem to be cropping up every day. Science is struggling to catch up. Since it is derived from a plant, CBD is a phytocannabinoid. Like plants, animals (including humans) also produce cannabinoids. They are called endocannabinoids. The ECS (endocannabinoid system) plays a role in several psychological and physiological processes, including memory and reproduction. When you ingest CBD, either as a capsule or a droplet, it interacts with your ECS to promote mental health. It especially shows a lot of promise when it comes to anxiety disorders such as PTSD and social anxiety. In one study, participants were given a CBD capsule before their public speaking task. The results showed a significant reduction in stress levels. In another study, volunteers were given CBD after taking THC. CBD reduced the anxiety effects that come with taking THC. Mallory Loflin, who is a psychologist at the University of California, said that reduction in anxiety only seems to be in people with anxiety pathology. So, it does not just dampen your central nervous system—it changes the pathological process. It is still not clear exactly how CBD reliefs anxiety. THC is known to cause anxiety, as well as promote drug-seeking behavior. Some experts have wondered whether CBD can dampen these behaviors. In one clinical trial study, CBD was given to people with heroin use disorder. After three days, they reported a significant drop in anxiety and lower levels of cortisol, the stress hormone. CBD also reduced drug carvings. Addiction is a craving disorder, according to Yasmin Hurd, a psychiatrist. The dampening effect of CBD on cravings can last a week after you take the last dose. And Hurd says that this represents a breakthrough. CBD is also providing some hope when it comes to schizophrenia. It reduces the severity of delusions and hallucinations when taken alongside an antipsychotic. Most of the successful clinical trials used daily CBD dosages ranging from 400 mg to 1000+ mg. This is way more than you can find in a commercial extract. Commercial capsules contain 10 to 25 mg each. Proper dosing has not been established yet. All CBD, whether derived from the hemp plant or marijuana plant, is the same and it is non intoxicating. Hemp is legal nationwide and hemp-derived CBD is sold in some stores. States that have legalized marijuana allow it to be sold in regulated dispensaries. Always ask your local dispensary where they sourced the CBD from. The FDA is expected to clarify more about CBD regulations soon.

Chapter Nine

CBD Salve: Everything You Need to Know

Cannabis plants such as marijuana and hemp contain many active cannabinoids. Industrial hemp is now legalized under the federal law. This has led to the cropping up of CBD salves and a ton of other CBD products. CBD (cannabidiol) is among the most active compounds in hemp plants. And it is known for its health benefits.

CBD oil has especially become quite popular in the health community. Unlike THC (tetrahydrocannabinol), CBD is not psychoactive. It does not have any intoxicating or euphoric effects on consumers. What Is CBD Salve? CBD-infused topicals include moisturizers, salves, oils, balms, and lotions with CBD as the main active ingredient. How can you safely use these topicals and salves? You must apply directly onto your skin and wait for it to absorb. It can help with skin conditions such as irritation, pain, and soreness. If the prescription is right and you use them properly, topical CBD products can be powerful. They can help with a lot of problems, from joint soreness to dermatitis. And they will not have the harsh side effects that chemical topicals have. The use of topical cannabis is nothing new. It can be traced back to ancient Egypt and Europe. People used them as treatment for inflamed muscles and skin as well as disinfectants. It is also possible that they were used as anesthetic. Now that CBD products seem to have re-emerged, people want to know how they can incorporate them into their day-to-day health routines. Most CBD-salves barely contain THC. The legal limit is 0.3%. They provide all the CBD health benefits, but without the intoxicating effects associated with cannabis. How Does a

CBD Salve Work? You apply CBD salves to the affected area. They relieve skin conditions such as itchiness, chronic pain, and soreness. Since the consumer does not ingest them, they do not go to the bloodstream directly. Instead, the skin layers absorb the product and retain it. The skin is capable of quickly absorbing water and other thin liquids. But it can also absorb lipid liquids with wax and oil. Once you apply the CBD salve, your skin begins the absorption process, and the healing starts. The salve, with its soothing properties, will relieve itchiness and pain. You can benefit from using CBD salves if you have psoriasis, dermatitis, and other skin conditions. CBD interacts with the endocannabinoid system (ECS) in the body. This system works to achieve homeostasis in the human body—this includes regulating how the skin responds to foreign substances. The receptors that make up the ECS control the body's immunity response, hormone regulation, skin sensitivity, response to pain, among other functions. When the CBD in salves starts working with the ECS receptors, you will start feeling the effects. Chronic joint pain is alleviated, any skin irritation is soothed and if your muscles are sore, they will start to relax. According to WHO (World Health Organization), CBD has no dependence or abuse potential. The legality of CBD is still a big issue. Some states have legalized it while others prohibit its production and consumption. Lotions and creams mainly differ with salves and balms when it comes to active ingredients and main bases. The same goes for CBD ointments. Creams and moisturizers contain some water and other moisturizing agents such as aloe vera. Salves and balms use lipids and fatty oils as well as wax. They can have little or no water. The difference is mainly in the texture and consistency. In terms of CBD content, salves and balms are different from lotions and creams. Read the labels keenly to know the potency. CBD salves can be used for localized muscle soreness, inflammation, tension, and skin discomfort. If you are looking for a natural solution to help you with pain, apply the salve to the affected area. It will help reduce irritation, inflammation or swelling. For topical conditions, direct application works best because the relief will be instantaneous. If you ingest CBD oil, it will take a while for you to start feeling the effects. Topicals work faster. Topicals do not also have to go through your digestive system. Tinctures, soft gels, and capsules are best used for physiological conditions such as migraines, insomnia, and anxiety. Rheumatoid arthritis affects many adults of all sizes and ages. When someone has arthritis, the connective tissue and joints in their body swell, causing acute discomfort and pain. It may also cause muscle and joint lock, making movement difficult.

Recent studies have shown that CBD has anti-inflammatory properties which may work to reduce arthritis symptoms such as swelling, inflammation and pain. Clinical trials have been successful. Other arthritis symptoms may include anxiety, sleep deprivation and difficulty relaxing. CBD as a dietary supplement can alleviate most of these symptoms. Most of the CBD products being sold will not be detectable on drug tests. Those that use CBD isolates (with pure CBD as the main active ingredient) are even less likely to show on drug tests. Full-spectrum products contain CBD and other cannabinoids, including THC, the psychoactive compound. If the THC level is high enough in your bloodstream, it may show on drug tests. But the legal THC level is 0.3%. It can barely test positive. If you take a heavy daily CBD dosage, it may show on a drug test. Cannabinoids (including THC) can accumulate in your body and be present for a few days. Talk to whoever is conducting the drug test about your CBD usage. Blosum's Herbal Botanical Salve is all-natural, vegan, and GMO-free. You will get free shipping and a discount if you are a first-time buyer. The salve is: Made in the USA, lab tested. Infused with ginger and turmeric essential oils. THC-free, 100% organic, 500 mg, CBD concentration, and Full-Spectrum CBD Salve. The Full-Spectrum Herbal Botanical Salve 500mg is commonly used for pain. Since it is a full-spectrum product, the CBD:THC ratio is healthy, and you benefit from the entourage effect.

The salve is: Made in the USA, lab-tested, Contains herbs like Vitamin E and Arnica Montana, Full-spectrum formulation, USDA certified organic, and 500 mg CBD concentration. Finding the right CBD salve is not easy. Always read the labels and buy from trustworthy sources.

Chapter Ten
CBD Capsules vs. CBD Oil

CBD products come in many different forms, as you will discover when researching CBD. CBD capsules and CBD oil tinctures are probably the most common. Do you get a better experience with CBD oils than with CBD capsules? And if you use capsules, is the cannabinoid amount per use the same as other methods? This article will answer all your questions to help you make an informed decision. CBD Oil Tincture: What Is It? You can say that CBD oil tinctures are the most common CBD products on the market today. One dropper can expose you to a full spectrum of cannabinoids and provide you with numerous health benefits. The extraction of CBD oil begins once the plant has been harvested. People use several extraction methods, including CO2 extraction. The result is a CBD oil containing cannabinoids. Plants are differently engineered, and so CBD oils may be different. Full-spectrum CBD oils will have many cannabinoids, but the THC level does not exceed 0.3% because of the federal law. Broad-spectrum CBD oils will also have most cannabinoids but no THC. Then there is CBD isolate which only contains one cannabinoid and that is CBD. The main advantage of CBD Oil Tinctures is quick absorption. One dropper under your tongue allows for quicker delivery and you will start feeling the effects within a short time. Additionally, droppers give you better control of your dosage. You can increase the serving amount if you do not feel any effects. And if the effects are too strong, you can reduce the serving. You do not have to buy a new bottle. CBD oil tinctures, however, can have a natural taste. It is "earthy" or "wood-like" and sometimes even flavorings cannot mask it. If you do not like this flavor, then that may prevent you from using tinctures. The other downside is that traveling can be tricky. You can get a lot of questions, especially if it is in your carry-on. A CBD Capsule: What Is It? CBD capsules are another easy way of taking CBD oil. But the process of making them is completely different from that of making CBD oil tinctures. CBD capsules are available in two forms: soft gel capsules containing CBD oil or soft gel capsules with powder-like CBD isolate. The methods of extraction are also different. CBD capsules are easy to use and discreet. You will not get any weird looks when taking a capsule. You can also take one with water and you will not have to worry about the natural flavor. If you choose to take CBD capsules, they will have to go through your digestive system. This means that the effects will not kick in immediately. Another thing, CBD capsules contain other agents like extra virgin oil and hemp oil. This may cause side effects. So read the label first to know all the ingredients. CBD Capsules Vs CBD Oil Tinctures: Which Is Better? This will depend on your attitude and personal preference. With tinctures you will feel the effects faster, but you may have to deal with the natural flavor. Capsules are convenient but the benefits take long to kick in.

Chapter Eleven
CBD Wax

Hemp-extracted CBD products are growing in popularity, and this includes CBD wax. More and more countries are now decriminalizing CBD use and easing their laws and regulations. People are starting to freely use the products for recreational and medical purposes. CBD wax is highly potent and commonly sought-after. What Is CBD Wax? It is a type of CBD concentrate, extracted from hemp. It does not contain psychotic compounds. It helps you get CBD benefits without the sedating side effects. Check out these amazing CBD wax facts. CBD Wax Comes in Different Types - Shatter: as you can guess from the name, CBD shatter looks like glass pieces. The texture is gooey, honey-like. Budder: this one is made by air pressure. Its texture is creamy, like butter. Crumble: the texture of this one is like that of feta cheese. The process of making it is the same as the one that is used for budder. Live resin: it is pricy, mainly because the extraction process is unique, and it is made using the freeze-dried method. Different Methods Are Used to Make CBD Wax - Butane Hash Oil (BHO) extraction: this is the most common process. Butane is the primary solvent used in the process. CO2 extraction: different types of trace cannabinols are extracted from the plant. Heat is then applied to make the potent compound. The resulting compound is cleaner compared to the one extracted using the BHO process. Anytime you want to buy hemp-extracted CBD wax, find a brand that is well-reviewed. Some, like Authentic Brands, even provide certificates of authenticity and safety certifications to show the extracted compounds and their potency. This cannabidiol concentrate provides instant results, unlike most of the other compounds derived from hemp.

It has a high cannabidiol content, which allows it to kick in and offer relief instantly. Many consumers go for this compound because of its high potency. It is highly effective and fast—which is what consumers want, really. Most people believe that dabbing high-concentrate CBD wax will have psychotic effects. But this could not be further from the truth. The concentrate does not have tetrahydrocannabinol or THC. This is the psychotic compound that gives users that high sensation. The fact that it does not contain THC makes CBD wax appropriate for use even during the day. Whether you are studying at home or busy at work, you can use CBD wax and get the benefits. You do not have to worry about getting high. Dabbing CBD Wax Comes with Many Benefits - Scientific research shows that this CBD concentrate can help with anxiety as well as chronic pain. It can also provide relief for arthritis patients. How Do You Use CBD Wax? CBD wax is mainly used in three main ways: by use of a bong, vaporizing and dabbing. Most people prefer dabbing. You can use nectar collectors (dab straws), dab pens or dab rigs. Vaporizing is a convenient way of ingesting CBD wax. You will need a vape pen for this.

Chapter Twelve
CBD Business

Were you thinking about launching a CBD business before COVID-19 struck? Has the pandemic made you think about expanding your business to include CBD? Whatever the case, now is a good time to dive into this quickly growing industry. It is expected to pass 20 billion within the next three years. And the number will continue to increase. So why should you join this market now? Since the pandemic began, wellness items went up 21.6% in sales, and this includes CBD. People are beginning to understand how important wellness is. They are keener about their health. Even before the pandemic, the sale of wellness products was still rising. The demand for organic products was up by 52%. Conventional products, on the other hand, have gone down 1% in sales pretty much every year for the past decade. Experts believe that the demand for natural products will go even higher post-pandemic. There is already a pattern in how people are shopping during the pandemic. Right before March last year, people stocked up on wellness and health supplies. The sale of vitamin supplements went up 1285% at the end of February, while that of food supplements went up 3117%. Sales dipped when people started settling into lockdown, but they began restocking again after a few weeks. eCommerce purchases, like health and wellness sales, have also increased. CBD businesses say that their online stores have been significant revenue sources. A brick-and-mortar store is beneficial but not a must. Most CBD businesses have decided to strictly stick to online stores. Integrating your business will not be that hard. eCommerce revenue has increased 37%. People are adding more products to their carts, and almost half of them are in the health and wellness category. It is unlikely that eCommerce purchases will go down post-pandemic. When it comes to food and beverage sales, demand for the following products has gone up: Melatonin, Curcumin, Medium-Chain Triglycerides (MCT) Oil, and Hemp/CBD. As more competition gets into the field, the options will increase. You can enter the blossoming CBD industry in two ways. First, there is the option of creating your own brand. You can decide to focus on a specific niche like women's fitness. And you will not have to compete with the promotions and sales of your supplier. The other option would be to buy wholesale. It is a cost-effective and easy method. How to Choose a CBD Source/ Supplier - See what clicks (look for a product that suits your brand). Third-party lab testing is important—you want to know what you are selling to your customers. Sample several products to see what resonates with you. Research the manufacturing facility, look for ISO, CoA and GMP certification. Partner with a good CBD source. They will offer the advice and guidance needed to navigate the industry. The CBD market is expected to hit $16.8 billion by 2025. CBD sellers have been diversifying sales channels to keep up with the increasing consumer demand. But CBD rules and regulations are still unclear, and this causes confusion. A CBD seller should fully understand the laws and create a clear fulfillment strategy for a smooth flow of things. Most sellers outsource to a dedicated fulfillment company (third-party logistics provider or 3PL). So here is all you need to know about that. Shipping CBD Is Legal, However... For CBD to be shippable and legal, it must meet certain criteria. It Should Be Hemp-Derived with Less Than 0.3% THC. Legal CBD, according to the Hemp Farming Act of 2018, is that which has been derived from hemp strands and contains less than 0.3% THC. The classification is legal in the 50 states and you can ship it across state lines. CBD from marijuana is only legal in several states and the regulations are different. The Seller Has to Source from a Licensed CBD Producer and Grower - You should have all the needed documentation to show that the grower and producer you are working with is licensed. You need a CoA (Certificate of Analysis) to show the level of THC, CBD, and other compounds in the product. USPS: to ship with them, you should have a state Department of Agriculture license showing authorization to produce hemp and the CBD should be hemp-derived with less than 0.3% hemp. UPS: the requirements are like those of USPS. But they will not ship hemp-products from a location that sells any marijuana products or marijuana. DHL: they require federal and state regulations compliance and the package being shipped should not have labeling or branding detailing the box contents. FedEx: marijuana- and hemp-derived CBD products are prohibited by FedEx. But some sellers have a written permission from FedEx to allow them to ship. Benefits of Third-Party Shipping - Low shipping costs. Reduced operating costs (you save on fulfilling essentials like labor, racking and rent) How to Choose a Shipping Partner - The fulfillment company must: Understand CBD Rules and Regulations. They should know what is legal when it comes to shipping and even storing CBD products. In case of new regulations or rules, they should be the ones alerting you. You also need to work with someone who can quickly resolve issues. eCommerce sales may be super high, but in-store retail sales are still higher. Urban Outfitters, Wholefoods, CVS, and other big names have started stocking CBD products. And more retailers will join the trend soon. The importance of working with a partner who can cooperate with retailers cannot be emphasized enough. Retailers can be strict, and you do not want to hurt the relationship. Provide Value-Added Services. You will need services like returns management, branded tape, custom knitting, and such services as your business grows. The legalization of cannabis has seen the market grow in terms of products, companies, and sales. This situation has captured the attention of investors since it appears to be a huge investment opportunity. Being a high risk and high growth investment, investors must approach it wisely. So here is a guide that you can use. Medical cannabis products: most states have legalized the use of medical cannabis. One needs to get a prescription from a specialist for conditions such as pain, stress, and anxiety. Adults use cannabis products: these are products that are mainly used for recreational purposes. Wellness uses cannabis: legislative texts don't recognize these products, but different marketing strategies are supporting it. Cannabis retailers and growers: these are companies that have outdoor facilities or greenhouses where they grow cannabis, harvest it and then distribute to end users. Cannabis-focused biotech: these are biotech companies that use cannabinoids to develop drugs. Auxiliary services and products suppliers in the supply chain: they offer raw materials such as packaging, pots, logistics, hydroponic systems, and lights to growers. Every investment comes with its degree of risk. Do not expect cannabis stocks to be any different. Here are the dangers involved. Political and legal risk: the political risk is diminishing because more countries are legalizing cannabis. But now, it is uncertain how exactly the industry will operate. Supply and demand imbalance: there are new players and new markets cropping up in the sector and the imbalances cause a high variability in profits and sales. Penny stocks: most of the titles are penny stocks. They are speculative, highly volatile and, historically, hard to trust. Financial risks: most companies follow a dominating-the-market strategy. This interferes with cash flows and profitability. Considerations for Finding a Stock - Research the strategy and management team of the company. - Understand the strategy and the competitive advantages it has. Prioritize a favorable financial situation— positive unit flows and low debt. How does the company acquire debt? For instance, raising capital through debt that is convertible into shares is risky. Assess the advantage in terms of production cost per gram. To control risk, you must first understand your risk profile. Define the base assumptions and terms with which you are making your decision. Cannabis companies have a short execution time of strategy and are volatile now which makes them high risk. Understand your options and establish an amount that you would be comfortable losing. Monitor the industry and the shares you acquire. Watch out for things that could have a positive effect like the federal government legalizing cannabis. With live investments, you invest in the company directly. But the liquidity risk is higher. However, if the business model works, they are super profitable. To find good projects, know the involved parties well and their strategy. There is a lot of potential in the quickly growing CBD industry. But the marketplace is crowded and creating a successful brand is not easy. The following tips highlight common mistakes and how to avoid them. They may not guarantee success, but they will help you launch efficiently and quickly. If you want your brand to be successful, you must be knowledgeable about CBD. You can start with Google searches, learn all there is to know about CBD. Look at its history, potential benefits, extraction processes, etc. Next, look for companies and experts in the field and talk to them. Take time to learn so you can finally make an informed decision when choosing a supplier. If you are determined to own a successful CBD business someday, you must start. While it is important to research first, some people spend so much time overanalyzing everything and holding themselves back. They want things to be perfect. In the end, they never start. Perfectionism can be an enemy of progress. You must move forward. Knowledge is important but you cannot learn everything at once. Start the business and you will learn more along the way. The name you pick for your business will affect a lot of things. CBD is still considered a high-risk business by some institutions. If you include words like cannabis, hemp or CBD, banks may not want to work with you. Your business name should not raise red flags. It should also provide room for expansion. A name like Lazarus Naturals is simple, easy to spell and easy to remember. It also allows for expansion into other natural products that do not naturally involve CBD. Once you have a name, the next step should be establishing an LLC. It is not an intimidating process as many people may think. It is not expensive either and it does not take a lot of time. Go to 99 Designs or Fiverr and look for a freelance designer to create a logo. This is another easy process. It is also a cheap way to get a high-quality logo design. Use Wix, Squarespace, or WordPress to create a website. They are inexpensive. Search Google for templates and look for a designer who can fill it with images and content. This is an especially important factor. When everything is high-quality, you will attract customers. More importantly, you will turn most of them into repeat customers. Finding a bank that will process CBD sales in the U.S can be stressful. There are very few people you can trust in the industry. Be careful to avoid falling into the hands of scammers. Look for a processor that does CBD sales and make sure they are based in the U.S. Coming up with your own formula may seem like a good idea. But you are better off sticking to what already sells best. Softgels and tinctures are quite popular right now and a safe bet. With time, you can try experimenting with unique products.

Conclusion

The legal cannabis industry has grown by 75% in its first year. This is just the beginning. It will continue to grow as more laws are made or revised in its favor. Some experts predict that the industry might be worth billions in the next five years. So, how can you earn money legally from marijuana? If you have a valuable skill set, finding a job in the industry will be easy. This could be sales, marketing, technology, accounting, design, and basically anything else that a business in the marijuana sector might need. There is also a high demand for ancillary positions. The marijuana market is strictly regulated, and this creates many new positions. In Colorado, you need a Support Badge to work with cannabis directly. You will pay $150 for this application but it will last a year. It certifies that you are not a cop or felon and are 21 years of age or older. For a managerial position where you must handle the product without being supervised, you will need a Key Badge. You will pay twice as much for this one and the application is extensive. There are countless high-level positions, but you can start with the entry-level ones such as growers, trimmers, manufacturers, and budtenders. Regardless of whether your state is weed-friendly, you can make some money from the industry through affiliate marketing or promoting another person's product in exchange for cash. The pay-off is usually a fraction of the proceeds. However, it could be in the form of other offers such as discounts etc. Just make sure you go through the fine print. To become an affiliate marketer, you need a website (it would be nice if it is in the marijuana niche) to post reviews, blog articles, and videos of the product. Next, focus on finding businesses with an affiliate market program then apply. When they approve you, you will get access to statistics and links to track important information. Finally, promote your website through forum discussions, email, and social media. Even better, use a business account rather than your personal account. Cannabis stocks may be the best way to invest any little money that you have. The financial risks here are higher than in other businesses because technically, the federal government can pull the plug on the cannabis industry any time. Regardless, the profits can be very lucrative. People are more than ready to invest their money in this industry because there are chances of making a big profit—and scammers know this. They will easily create "companies" to tempt you into buying. When the share prices peak, the scammers will sell for a tremendous profit and leave the investors with stocks worth nothing. Companies like MarijuanaStocks.com make the trade easier. You will find all the up-to-date stock information here. Before investing in a company, do a lot of research and know everything about it. Pain affects so many Americans—much more than heart disease, diabetes and cancer combined. This is according to a study by Elsevier. A third of those with pain experiences say that it affects their daily lives and is often disabling. People with acute and/or chronic pain desire to find an effective but safe way of managing the pain. Opioids, NSAIDs (non-steroidal anti-inflammatory drugs) and acetaminophen are the most common painkillers. However, most of them will either lead to dependency or have side effects when used for long. CBD (cannabidiol) oil is quickly becoming a popular alternative to pain relievers. CBD reduces pain by alleviating inflammation in your body. Many industries are slowly fading, but there is one that has continued to grow tremendously over the past few years—the marijuana industry. More states continue to legalize and tax each day. With the business booming there is a lot of money to be gained in the cannabis industry. The state of Colorado, for instance, reported $1+ billion in sales in just eight months. It is not guaranteed that everyone who decides to sell cannabis is going to become rich instantly. However, there is plenty of marijuana money available. Experts in this industry, lucky for you, have some tips to help you make the best of this opportunity. Here is advice from the experts. President of SinglePoint, Wil Ralston: he says that the cannabis industry is perfect for making money. According to him, there are so many opportunities for entrepreneurship or offering ancillary business services such as web design and marketing. Another way to make huge profits is by investing. Cannabis-eccentric companies offer a myriad of opportunities for investment. If you are paying attention, you will notice that there are companies that are looking to be funded in the cannabis industry. COO of Marimed Inc. Timothy Shaw: he believes in creating a reputable brand identity; one that patients can always rely on for purity, precision dosage, and consistency. A high-quality brand is an essential ingredient for success in a cannabis business. Your brand should convey an authentic story and be relevant to the needs of your customers for more income. Founder of Feuerstein Kulick LLP, Mitchell Kulick: the cannabis industry is not different from other industries in the U.S. Therefore, you have a chance of making money as an operator or entrepreneur. It is harder than many portray it to be and there are no guarantees. You can also develop a business that works to support operators by offering payroll solutions, point-of-sale-software systems, advertising platforms, legal services, etc. Whichever area you choose, be prepared to face hurdles worse than those that run fully legal businesses. Kulick hopes that the risks and complications of the marijuana market will bring tremendous rewards to those who decide to work hard and build this industry. Founder of Terra Tech, Derek Peterson: entrepreneurs and pioneers alike are eager to make some cash in the most lucrative ways. Peterson says that he has been doing this for more than seven years and the one thing that is more important than anything else is patience. It does not matter what area you choose; you must be patient. You will not become wealthy overnight in the marijuana industry. There are everyday challenges. It is also not a legal business federally so if you are interested, you need to be ready to stay. CEO of Burn TV, Jason Santos: Santos says that the cannabis industry is even more interesting because it creates so many opportunities other than those of cannabis-based products. There is the ancillary sector that he thinks is more lucrative and attractive. It also has fewer legal restrictions. For anyone looking to get into the cannabis industry, Santos highly recommends the business services line. For this limited time, cannabis businesses have a chance to become major players in smaller ponds. How can they do this? By specializing and being great at a certain thing. The cannabis product market is diverse. If you ask most people, they will tell you that cannabis is just a flower for smoking. Nonetheless, this is a small part of it. Of course, many cannabis extracts can be dabbed, vaped, or smoked. But you will find that manufactured cannabis products like transdermal patches, beverages, brownies, and gummies make up half of the market. In some states, their sales growth is off the charts. There are thousands of compliance consultants, lawyers, and software developers that offer their support behind the scenes. As an entrepreneur, you have countless areas to create a mark but there is the temptation to try it all. Today, most cannabis companies are mainly left to grow leisurely since interstate commerce does not exist to bring in competition. Most consumers get their cannabis products from local shops. Those in prohibition states go to free states to try out legal cannabis. If the federal government legalizes cannabis, allowing interstate distribution, incumbent businesses will find it harder to compete for customers with the bigger multinational corporations. As soon as the smaller ponds merge into one ocean, the bigger fish will begin to swim in. Cannabis businesses will either find a small pond and become king there or learn to swim like sharks. Businesses in many industries typically prefer to find one thing and specialize. You do not see grocery stores making their own ketchup or growing their own vegetables. However, it is common to see a cannabis business combining retail, distribution, processing, and cultivation into a single organization. Oversupply will cause prices to fall. A producer merges with a retail store that carries their product exclusively to steady demand and secure great prices. Doing everything on your own may increase costs and, consequently, the final price. Customers will choose to buy the same product at a lower price somewhere else. Your other option will be to lower prices and suffer losses. If you are an aspiring entrepreneur or business owner, find something you are good at and be the best. Dominating a niche before a huge corporation gets involved may make your business valuable enough to be bought. You can even do well enough and become the one that is acquiring businesses. Whatever you do, the rewards will be greater if you focus on what you are best at. More cannabidiol applications are being introduced to the market across different industries such as pharmaceuticals, skin care, pet products, food and beverage, health products, and cosmetics. Therefore, sales in the CBD market are expected to go beyond $20 billion by 2024, in the United States alone. This is according to ArcView Market Research and BDS Analytics. The prediction includes all products such as those sold through pharmaceuticals, licensed dispensaries, and the general market retail, that is, mass merchants, pharmacies, grocery stores, smoke shops and cafes. The figure came from the proprietary data sets of BDS analytics. It offers a deeper understanding of both the history and evolution of consumer behavior, pricing, purchasing and assortment of the cannabis product. Afterwards, this was expanded with insights and integral data sets from data partners. BDS Analytics is already a reputable data provider in the cannabis industry. Now it aims at offering quality insights to CBD market decision makers through its very own CBD Market Monitor service. BDS Analytics Co-Founder and CEO, Roy Bingham, says that CBD is growing from a subcategory of cannabis to a fully independent industry. According to their growth forecast, all distribution channels considered, the compound annual growth rate is expected to be 49% by 2024. For anyone involved in the industry, this is an amazing opportunity. However, it also means that decisions down the road must be made using the best data. It is also predicted that most of the CBD sales will likely happen in general stores and not cannabis dispensaries. This is because major retailers are announcing their private label development and stocking of the products. BDS Analytics goes on to predict that CBD products' success depends on consistent labeling, dosing, and education. There are two reasons why BDS Analytics thinks that CBD is better off compared to supplement and nutraceutical ingredients: 1) it has a well-documented history of wellness and health use and 2) there is scientific evidence to back some of its claims. Consumers are becoming more interested in ingestible/edibles (food, beverages, pills, tinctures) and topicals (salves, balms, creams). Sales in CBD have exploded over the past few months. However, the Vice President of Consumer Insights, Jessica Lukas thinks that there is a long way to go. Many have no idea of the difference between CBD and THC. Therefore, BDS is determined to continue offering in-depth data. They aspire to inform and guide a new but booming industry. Here is what a comprehensive sample of BDS Analytics data concerning CBD contains: An expected compound annual rate of 49%. A total market value of $45 billion by 2024 (for both CBD and THC products). Dispensary CBD sales are growing at a higher rate than overall dispensary sales. Dispensary CBD sales clearly indicate the direction of the general market for CBD products. The average CBD consumer is aged 40, employed full time and has a higher education. BDS Analytics offers more information on their website. The time is now to invest in the cannabis green rush. Dr. Sanjay Gupta, in a *The Doctor Oz Show* segment, explained why some people can take several CBD gummies and feel nothing at all. He said that if you want to feel any kind of effect you will have to take hundreds of milligrams. The CBD products you buy over the counter will only have about 2 to 22 milligrams of CBD. CBD stands for cannabidiol—a compound found hemp and marijuana. Marijuana also contains tetrahydrocannabinol, or CBD. This is the chemical that gives a user a "high". Hemp, on the other hand, contains less than 0.3% of THC. Simply put, both marijuana and hemp contain CBD, but the CBD in hemp lacks THC so it cannot get you high. Even before CBD was legal according to federal law, the FDA had already approved it.

Hemp was legalized in 2018 after the Farm Bill was passed and, consequently, the CBD in it was also legalized. The laws are still somewhat unclear, but Dr. Oz and Dr. Gupta both believe that the authorities will not come looking for you because of CBD possession. The confusion is even more when it comes to state laws. Authorities seem to be dealing with CBD based on specific cases. A woman was arrested in Disney World for CBD oil possession in 2019. But she was released after producing a doctor's note. Brooke Alpert, *CBD Snapshot* editor and cannabis practitioner, believes that this is because there is still so much confusion when it comes to CBD. Since you can buy hemp CBD legally over the counter, most people do not bother to get a doctor's note. In the case of medical marijuana, you will need a doctor's note unless the state you are in has legalized it. With more questions about CBD than answers, here are key things you should know. The CBD craze began with what has come to be referred to as "Charlotte's Web", according to Dr. Gupta. Charlotte, a little girl, was having seizures. Her mother, having tried different solutions in vain, decided to give CBD a try. After taking CBD oil, Charlotte went from having 300 seizures to having none—in only one week! This got the FDA interested. And after five years, they approved a CBD prescription drug, Epidiolex, for epilepsy. Is the Opioid Epidemic Coming to an End? In states where CBD has been legalized, opioid prescription rates have noticeably declined. The opioid epidemic does not look like it will end any time soon. So, doctors are watching CBD closely to see how it can help them change painkiller prescriptions. Marijuana has shown to help with treating chronic pain. Dr. Gupta also says that some PTSD patients claim that CBD has greatly helped change their lives. What's Next for CBD? Both Dr. Oz and Dr. Gupta have called for more research about CBD so Americans battling medical issues can find a solution.